The Low-FODMAP Diet Cookbook

The low-FODMAP diet step by step: a personalized plan to relieve symptoms of IBS and other digestive disorders - with deliciously satisfying recipes

TABLE OF CONTENTS

The information in the following pages is broadly considered a truthful and accurate account of facts and as such, any inattention, use, or misuse of the information in question by the reader will render any resulting actions solely under their purview. There are no scenarios in which the publisher or the original author of this work can be in any fashion deemed liable for any hardship or damages that may befall them after undertaking information described herein.

Additionally, the information in the following pages is intended only for informational purposes and should thus be thought of as universal. As befitting its nature, it is presented without assurance regarding its prolonged validity or interim quality. Trademarks that are mentioned are done without written consent and can in no way be considered an endorsement from the trademark holder.

BREAKFAST RECIPES

Hash Brown Egg Nests

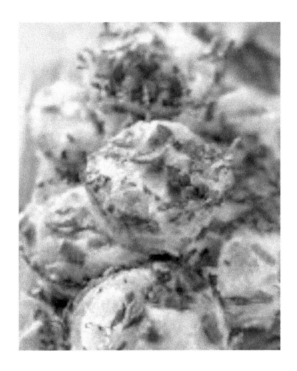

Preparation Time: 15 minutes

Cooking Time: 25 minutes

Servings: 2

Ingredients:

- 2 cups shredded hash brown potatoes, uncooked, drain liquid if present
- ½ tablespoon garlic infused oil or plain olive oil
- 1 small zucchini or summer squash, trimmed, very thinly sliced
- 3 slices bacon, cooked, cut into bite size pieces
- 1 egg white
- 6 large eggs
- Salt to taste
- Pepper to taste
- A handful fresh parsley, chopped
- 1 small bell pepper, chopped
- Oil, to grease

Directions:

1. Grease a 6-count muffin tin with a generous amount of oil.
2. Add potatoes, garlic oil, salt and pepper into a bowl.
3. Add egg white and fold gently.
4. Divide the mixture into the muffin cups. Press it on to the bottom as well as the sides of the cup.
5. To your preheated oven at 425 °F bake it for 15 minutes.

---

6. Place a few slices of squash in each of the cups, over the potato crust.
7. Sprinkle some cheese.
8. Crack an egg into each cup. Place bacon pieces on top.
9. Bake until the way you like the eggs cooked.
10. Sprinkle parsley and bell pepper on top and serve.

Nutrition: Calories: 150 Carbs: 15g Fat: 9g Protein: 1g

Sweet Potato & Eggs, Sunny Side up

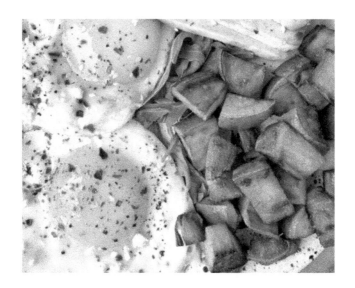

Preparation Time: 10 minutes

Cooking Time: 25 minutes

Servings: 4

Ingredients:

- 2 cups sweet potatoes, thinly sliced, with its skin
- 4 large eggs
- Salt to taste
- Pepper to taste
- 2 teaspoons olive oil
- ½ cup baby spinach or kale, sliced

Directions:

1. Place a skillet over medium heat. Add the oil. When the oil is heated, make 2 discs of sweet potatoes using ¼ cup for each disc. If your pan is large enough, you can make all the 4 at once.
2. Cook until the underside is light brown. Flip sides and cook the other side until light brown.
3. Crack an egg on each potato disc. Cover the pan and lower heat. Cook until eggs are cooked as per your desire.
4. Sprinkle spinach, salt and pepper.
5. Slide on to a plate and serve.

Nutrition: Calories: 150 Carbs: 1g Fat: 10g Protein: 13g

Berry Lime Coconut Smoothie

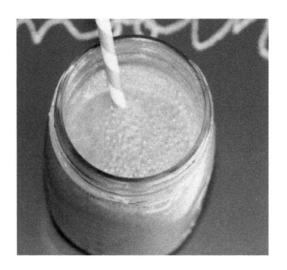

Preparation Time: 10 minutes

Cooking Time: 0 minute

Servings: 2

Ingredients:

- 1 cup berries of your choice, fresh or frozen
- 4 tablespoons fresh lime juice
- 2 teaspoons chia seeds
- Ice, to be used if using fresh berries
- 4 tablespoons flaked coconut
- 8 ounces plain non-fat lactose free yogurt
- ¼ cup water

Directions:

1. Add berries, lime juice, chia seeds, ice, coconut, yogurt and water into a blender and blend until smooth.
2. Pour into tall glasses and serve.

Nutrition: Calories: 230 Carbs: 52g Fat: 2g Protein: 2g

Tropical Passion Smoothie

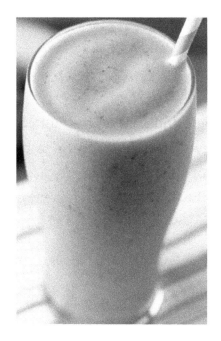

Preparation Time: 10 minutes

Cooking Time: 0 minute

Servings: 2

Ingredients:

- 1 passion fruit, chopped
- 1 cup frozen pineapple
- ¼ cup coconut milk
- 1 cup dairy free milk

Directions:

1. Add pineapple and passion fruit into a freezer safe bag. Freeze until you need to make the smoothie.
2. Empty the contents of the bag into a blender.
3. Add rest of the ingredients and blend until smooth.
4. Pour into glasses and serve.

Nutrition: Calories: 216 Carbs: 51g Fat: 4g Protein: 3g

Banana 'N' Peanut Butter Smoothie

Preparation Time: 10 minutes

Cooking Time: 0 minute

Servings: 2

Ingredients:

- 2 bananas, peeled, sliced, frozen
- 3-4 tablespoons natural peanut butter
- 1 cup almond milk
- Ice cubes, as required

Directions:

1. Add the banana, peanut butter, almond milk and ice cubes into a blender and blend until smooth.
2. Pour into tall glasses and serve.

Nutrition: Calories: 253 Carbs: 35g Fat: 8g Protein: 15g

Blueberry Kiwi Smoothie with a Hit of Mint

Preparation Time: 10 minutes

Cooking Time: 0 minute

Servings: 2

Ingredients:

- 1 cup frozen blueberries
- 2/3 cup lactose free yogurt
- A handful fresh mint leaves (12-15 leaves)
- 2 kiwifruits, peeled, chopped
- 2/3 cup water

Directions:

1. Add the blueberries, yogurt, mint leaves, water and kiwifruits into a blender and blend until smooth.
2. Pour into tall glasses and serve.

Nutrition: Calories: 218 Carbs: 46g Fat: 0g Protein: 4g

Mixed Fruit Smoothie

Preparation Time: 10 minutes

Cooking Time: 0 minute

Servings: 2

Ingredients:

- 2 cups frozen mixed fruits of your choice
- ¼ cup light coconut milk
- ¼ teaspoon lemon zest, grated (optional)
- A handful walnuts, finely chopped, to top
- ¼ cup lemon Chobani yogurt or lactose free yogurt of your choice
- Water, as required, to dilute
- 4 teaspoons shredded coconut, to top

Directions:

1. Mix all the ingredients into a blender and blend until smooth.
2. Pour into tall glasses. Sprinkle coconut and walnuts on top and serve.

Nutrition: Calories: 70 Carbs: 15g Fat: 0g Protein: 1g

Pumpkin Smoothie

Preparation Time: 10 minutes

Cooking Time: 0 minute

Servings: 2

Ingredients:

- 1 medium ripe banana, peeled, sliced, frozen
- 1 cup canned coconut milk
- 2 tablespoons maple syrup
- ¼ teaspoon ground cinnamon
- ½ cup canned pumpkin puree
- ½ teaspoon pumpkin pie spice
- 1 cup ice

Directions:

1. Transfer all your ingredients into a blender and blend until smooth.
2. Pour into tall glasses and serve.

Nutrition: Calories: 200 Carbs: 19g Fat: 4g Protein: 21g

LUNCH RECIPES

Slow Cooker Chicken Rice Soup

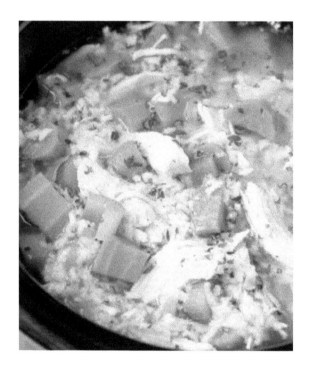

Preparation Time: 15 minutes

Cooking Time: 8 hours

Servings: 4

Ingredients:

- 4 medium carrots, peeled & chopped
- 1 courgette, chopped
- 1lb boneless, skinless chicken breasts
- 15g/½oz butter
- ½ teaspoon dried thyme
- 175g/6oz brown rice
- 1lt/4 cups gluten free, low FodMap chicken stock
- 250ml/1 cup water
- 2 teaspoon olive oil
- 1 small leek, green parts only, sliced
- Juice from 1 lemon
- Salt & pepper
- 1 tablespoon Parmesan cheese, grated
- 4 sprigs parsley to garnish

Directions:

1. Tip the carrots, courgette, chicken breasts, butter, thyme, and rice into your slow cooker. Pour in the stock and the water. Put a lid to it and cook on Low for 8 hours or on High for 4.
2. Remove the chicken breasts to a chopping board and turn the slow cooker up to High if necessary.

3. Heat the oil in a frying pan. Sauté the leek for about 8 minutes, until tender.
4. Prick to pieces the chicken with two forks and return it to the slow cooker. Stir in the leeks, then cover and cook for a few minutes until the chicken is heated through.
5. Turn off the slow cooker before you stir in the lemon juice. Season the soup with salt and pepper to taste. If you don't have a slow cooker, just use an ordinary large pan. Omit the water and cook for 30-45 minutes instead of 4 or 8 hours.

Nutrition: Calories: 321 Carbs: 45g Fat: 5g Protein: 0g

Butternut Squash Salad

Preparation Time: 10 minutes

Cooking Time: 0 minute

Servings: 6

Ingredients:

- 600g/1lb5oz butternut squash, peeled, deseeded chopped
- 2 teaspoons olive oil, + 2 tablespoons
- 2 teaspoons sesame seeds
- 1 tablespoon fresh lemon juice
- 3 teaspoons brown sugar
- 2 teaspoons wholegrain mustard
- 150g/5oz spinach leaves
- 75g/3oz toasted pine nuts
- Salt & pepper

Directions:

1. Preheat the oven to 220C/430F/Gas7. Line a baking tray with greaseproof paper.
2. Tip the squash into a large bowl. Sprinkle some, and season well with salt and pepper. Toss the squash until evenly coated in the oil. Arrange it on the baking tray in a single layer.
3. Bake in the oven for 25-30 minutes or until golden brown, turning once half way through cooking.

4. Remove the tray from the oven and scatter the sesame seeds evenly over the squash. Go back it to the oven and bake for 5 more minutes, until the seeds are lightly toasted. Remove from oven and set aside to cool.
5. In a bowl, whisk together the lemon juice, 2 tablespoons olive oil, mustard and brown sugar. Season with salt and pepper.
6. Tip the squash into a bowl. Add the spinach and pine nuts and drizzle the dressing over the top. Toss until everything is coated in the dressing.
7. Serve at once. Enjoy this on its own for lunch, or serve as a side dish with dinner.

Nutrition: Calories: 568 Carbs: 53g Fat: 39g Protein: 11g

Shrimp Salad

Preparation Time: 15 minutes

Cooking Time: 15 minutes

Servings: 4

Ingredients:

- 250g/9oz shrimp, peeled and cooked
- 1 tablespoon olive oil
- 500g/1lb 2oz brown rice, cooked weight
- 100g/3½oz cucumber, peeled & chopped
- ½ red pepper, deseeded & chopped
- 125g/4oz green beans, finely sliced
- 75g/3oz feta cheese, crumbled
- Salt & pepper
- 2 tablespoons extra virgin olive oil
- 2 tablespoons red wine vinegar
- 3 tablespoons fresh basil, chopped, + more to garnish
- 3 tablespoons fresh parsley, chopped, + more to garnish

Directions:

1. Heat the olive oil in a frying pan, and fry the shrimp for about 3-5 minutes, until cooked.
2. Meanwhile, in a large bowl, mix together the rice, cucumber, red pepper, beans and feta. Using a small bowl, whisk together the extra virgin olive oil, red wine

vinegar, basil and parsley. Drizzle this dressing over the salad and toss to combine.

3. Divide the salad into 4 serving bowls and place the cooked shrimp on top. Garnish with freshly chopped basil and parsley leaves.

4. A treat to take to work, or to serve to friends at a lunch party.

Nutrition: Calories: 330 Carbs: 19g Fat: 20g Protein: 21g

Butternut Squash and Lemon Risotto

Preparation Time: 15 minutes

Cooking Time: 35 minute

Servings: 4

Ingredients:

- 250g/9oz butternut squash, peeled, deseeded & chopped
- 2 large carrots, peeled & chopped
- 2 tablespoons olive oil
- Salt & pepper
- 300g/11oz Arborio rice
- 50g/2oz leek, green parts only, finely chopped
- 1 tablespoon garlic infused olive oil
- 1 tablespoon olive oil
- 1lt/4 cups gluten free, low FodMap chicken stock
- 2 lemons, to yield 1 teaspoon lemon zest & 2½ tablespoon juice
- 165g/5½oz spinach, finely chopped
- 3 tablespoons fresh coriander, chopped
- 50g/2oz Parmesan cheese, grated

Directions:

1. Preheat the oven to 200C/400F/Gas6.
2. Place the squash and the carrot on a baking tray in a single layer, and drizzle with 1 tablespoon olive oil. Season with salt and pepper.

---

3. Bake your vegetables for about 20-25 minutes until the vegetables are soft and lightly golden. Stir them up once or twice during cooking.
4. Meanwhile, heat 1 tablespoon olive oil and the garlic infused oil together in a large pan, and fry the leek for a couple of minutes. Mix in the rice and cook gently for another minute.
5. Gradually pour in the chicken stock, a little at a time, allowing the rice to absorb it before adding more. Stir frequently.
6. When the rice is cooked and the stock absorbed, stir in the spinach, lemon juice and lemon zest. Season with salt and pepper to taste. Stir in the roasted squash and carrots, the coriander and the Parmesan. Serve and enjoy.

Nutrition: Calories: 378 Carbs: 64g Fat: 10g Protein: 6g

Spicy Steak Salad

Preparation Time: 15 minutes

Cooking Time: 15 minute

Servings: 4

Ingredients:

- 2 teaspoons Lebanese spice mix
- 500g/1lb 2oz beef sirloin steaks
- Olive oil cooking spray
- 1 romaine lettuce, roughly chopped
- 2 medium tomatoes, roughly chopped
- 1 cucumber, roughly chopped
- 1 red pepper, deseeded & chopped
- 16 large olives, pitted & halved
- 1 tablespoons red wine vinegar
- 1 teaspoons Dijon mustard

Directions:

1. Rub the Baharat spices into both sides of the steaks.
2. Heat a frying pan and spray it with olive oil. Place the steaks in the pan and cook for a minute or two on each side, until they're cooked to your preference.
3. Remove them from the pan and set them aside on a plate to rest for a few minutes.
4. Meanwhile, arrange the lettuce, tomatoes, cucumber, pepper and olives on 4 plates.

5. Using a small bowl, whisk together the extra virgin olive oil, vinegar and mustard.
6. Slice the steaks thinly and arrange it over the salad on each plate.
7. Drizzle the olive oil dressing over the top, and serve at once.

Nutrition: Calories: 535 Carbs: 70g Fat: 14g Protein: 35g

Stuffed Red Pepper

Preparation Time: 15 minutes

Cooking Time: 25 minutes

Servings: 1

Ingredients:

- Olive oil cooking spray
- 1 red pepper, deseeded & halved
- 50g/2oz cooked leftover chicken, shredded
- 2 tomatoes, chopped
- 2 basil leaves, torn
- Salt & pepper
- 25g/1oz mozzarella cheese, chopped
- 1 tablespoon Parmesan cheese, grated
- Chopped parsley to garnish

Directions:

1. Preheat the oven to 200C. Line a baking tray with parchment. Spray the parchment with oil.
2. Place the pepper halves on the baking tray, cut sides upwards. Divide the chicken between the two halves.
3. Mix the tomatoes and basil together in a bowl. Season with salt and pepper. Spoon this mixture over the chicken in the pepper halves.

4. Scatter the mozzarella evenly into the halves, then sprinkle on the Parmesan. Grind on a little more black pepper.
5. In the oven put your pepper and bake it for about 20 minutes, until the pepper halves are soft.
6. Serve and enjoy.

Nutrition: Calories: 128 Carbs: 6g Fat: 11g Protein: 26g

Bacon and Brie Frittata

Preparation Time: 10 minutes

Cooking Time: 20 minutes

Servings: 4

Ingredients:

- 1 tablespoon olive oil
- 8 rashers smoked bacon
- 6 eggs, lightly beaten
- 1 tablespoon chives, chopped
- Freshly ground black pepper, to taste
- 100g/3½oz Brie cheese, sliced

Directions:

1. Preheat the grill.
2. Using a small pan, heat your half of the olive oil. Fry the bacon until it's crispy. Drain it on kitchen towel.
3. Also the remaining oil heat it in the same pan. Using bowl, mix the eggs together with the bacon, chives and black pepper. Pour the egg mixture into the frying pan and cook over a low heat until it begins to set.
4. Lay the Brie on top of the setting egg, then slide the pan under the grill until the egg is set and golden.
5. Take it from the pan and cut into wedges just before serving.
6. Enjoy with crunchy salad and gluten-free toast.

Nutrition: Calories: 327 Carbs: 2g Fat: 26g Protein: 17g

Easy Chicken and Cranberry Sandwich

Preparation Time: 10 minutes

Cooking Time: 0 minute

Servings: 2

Ingredients:

- 350g/12oz cooked chicken breasts, shredded
- 3 tablespoons mayonnaise
- 1 tablespoon cranberry sauce
- Handful rocket
- 4 slices gluten free bread, spread with non-dairy spread.

Directions:

1. Combine the chicken and mayonnaise together in a bowl.
2. Divide it between two slices of bread. Top with the rocket and some cranberry sauce.
3. Close the sandwiches and enjoy.
4. Use other salad greens instead of rocket if you prefer. Or use leftover turkey instead of chicken and make a delicious Christmas sandwich

Nutrition: Calories: 230 Carbs: 25g Fat: 7g Protein: 16g

Chicken Wraps

Preparation Time: 10 minutes

Cooking Time: 20 minutes

Servings: 4

Ingredients:

- ½ cucumber, halved & sliced
- 1 small carrot, peeled & grated
- 1 tablespoon white wine vinegar
- 2 tablespoons vegetable oil
- 8 boneless, skinless chicken thighs, sliced
- 1 teaspoon freshly grated ginger
- 3 tablespoons light brown soft sugar
- 2 tablespoons gluten free soy sauce
- 120ml/½ cup water
- 8 small gluten free wraps
- 2 Little Gem lettuces, leaves separated and halved

Directions:

1. Using a small bowl, mix the cucumber, carrot and white wine vinegar. Set aside.
2. Using a frying pan heat your oil, and fry the chicken until it's fully cooked and golden brown. Remove to a plate and set aside.
3. Reduce the heat and warm the rest of the oil in the pan. Fry the ginger for about 2 minutes until it's softened.

Add the sugar, soy sauce and water. Bring to the boil and let it cook for 5 minutes or so until it forms into a sauce.

4. Return the chicken to the pan and heat through.

5. Warm the wraps according to the packet instructions. Spread them on 4 plates. Arrange the lettuce on each, then the chicken mixture, and the cucumber and carrot.

6. Make sure you use low FodMap wraps to avoid irritable ingredients.

Nutrition: Calories: 178 Carbs: 18g Fat: 4g Protein: 16g

DINNER RECIPES

Spinach Artichoke Hummus Dip

Preparation Time: 10 minutes

Cooking Time: 30 minutes

Servings: 10

Ingredients:

- 10 ounces Roasted Red Pepper Hummus or Regular hummus (We used Sabra)
- 1/3 cup plain Greek Style yogurt
- 2 garlic cloves (1 teaspoon minced)
- ½ cup parmesan crumbles or shredded
- 1 cup spinach leaves
- 4 artichoke hearts
- 3 basil leaves
- ½ small Lemon - juice
- 1 teaspoon Salt and pepper to taste
- Some Olive oil

Directions:

1. Ready to preheat the oven to 400 degrees F. Lightly grease an 8-inch square baking dish.

2. Combine the hummus, yogurt, artichoke, basil, spinach, artichoke hearts, ½ the lemon, salt, pepper and garlic in a food processor.
3. Puree.
4. Add 1/3 cup parmesan and puree.
5. Add a little olive oil and seasoning to taste.
6. Pour into the prepared dish.
7. Sprinkle on the remaining parmesan.
8. Bake, covered, for 20 minutes.
9. Take off its lid and bake for an additional 10 minutes.
10. Broil for 1 minute to get the top nicely browned.
11. Top with herbs, spinach, pepper, lemon slices and a little olive oil and parmesan before serving.
12. Serve with veggies or crackers.

Nutrition: Calories: 70 Carbs: 4g Fat: 6g Protein: 1g

Strawberry Basil Quinoa Salad

Preparation Time: 10 minutes

Cooking Time: 0 minute

Servings: 4

Ingredients:

- For the champagne vinaigrette
- ½ cup extra-virgin olive oil
- ¼ cup champagne vinegar (you can substitute balsamic, apple cider or even red wine vinegar)
- 2 tablespoons honey
- 1 tablespoon Dijon mustard
- Pinch of salt and pepper to taste
- For the salad
- 1 cup quinoa, cooked
- 1 cup fresh strawberries, sliced
- ½ cup crumbled feta cheese (goat cheese is a good substitute)
- 4 cups fresh baby spinach, finely chopped (you can also use arugula)
- 1 small bunch fresh basil, very thinly sliced
- 1 small avocado, diced
- Pine nuts or sesame seeds for garnish (optional)

Directions:

1. Combine the vinaigrette ingredients in the blender and blend until smooth.
2. Combine all ingredients, except feta and pine nuts in a bowl and mix well.
3. Serve immediately, garnished with the feta and pine nuts.

Nutrition: Calories: 250 Carbs: 25g Fat: 10g Protein: 15g

Strawberry Lemon Popsicles

Preparation Time: 5 minutes

Cooking Time: 0 minute

Servings: 4

Ingredients:

- ½ cup lemon tea or water
- ½ cup strawberry pieces
- 1 tablespoon fresh lemon juice
- 1 tablespoon white sugar
- 2 teaspoons chia seeds
- 2 tablespoon strawberry slices (optional to add)

Directions:

1. Combine the tea or water, strawberries, lemon juice, sugar and chia seeds in a blender.
2. Blend until smooth.
3. If desired, add in additional strawberry slices after blending so there are small pieces of fruit in the popsicles.
4. Fill Popsicle molds about ¾ full.
5. Freeze until solid, about 3-4 hours.
6. Remove from the mold and serve cold.

Nutrition: Calories: 170 Carbs: 22g Fat: 12g Protein: 2g

Strawberry Lemonade

Preparation Time: 5 minutes

Cooking Time: 0 minute

Servings: 2

Ingredients:

- 1.5 cup strong lemon tea (make sure it is low FODMAP, such as rooibos)
- ¾ cup frozen strawberries
- 1 tablespoon fresh lemon juice
- 1 tablespoon white sugar or maple syrup
- ½ cup ice cubes optional
- Plus extra strawberries and/or lemon slices for garnish

Directions:

1. Combine the tea, strawberries, lemon juice, and sugar and ice cubes, if desired, to a blender.
2. Blend well.
3. Season to taste.
4. Serve chilled.

Nutrition: Calories: 60 Carbs: 15g Fat: 0g Protein: 0g

Sushi Bowls

Preparation Time: 15 minutes

Cooking Time: 5 minutes

Servings: 4

Ingredients:

- 2 teaspoons rice vinegar
- 2 teaspoons sugar
- 2 cups cooked brown rice (or other favorite)
- 1 pound smoked salmon, sliced into bite sized pieces
- 1 cucumber, julienned
- 2 carrots, julienned
- ½ avocado, sliced* (optional)
- 1 nori sheet, sliced
- 2 teaspoon wasabi powder
- 1 teaspoon water
- 3 tablespoons mayonnaise
- Toasted sesame seeds
- Low sodium tamari (or coconut amino)

Directions:

1. Whisk together the vinegar and sugar. Add the brown rice and mix well.
2. Evenly divide between four bowls.
3. Top the rice with an equal portion of the salmon, cucumber, carrot, avocado and nori.

---

4. Mix the wasabi and water until a paste is formed, then add the mayonnaise and mix well.
5. Top the salmon and rice with a drizzle of the wasabi and garnish with sesame seeds.
6. Serve immediately with tamari.

Nutrition: Calories: 500 Carbs: 55g Fat: 23g Protein: 20g

VEGETABLES, SOUP AND SALADS RECIPES

Minestrone Soup

Preparation Time: 20 minutes

Cooking Time: 25 minutes

Servings: 4

Ingredients

- 80g smoked pancetta, finely chopped
- 1 potato, medium, peeled & diced into 1cm cubes
- 2 carrots, diced finely
- 1 zucchini, diced finely
- Approximately 5 cups boiling water
- 1 tin of tomatoes, chopped
- A good pinch of pepper and salt
- 1 celery stick, sliced finely
- A handful of fresh basil leaves, torn or chopped roughly
- 1 heaped tablespoon of rice
- A large handful of grated Parmesan cheese
- 1 tablespoon garlic flavored olive oil plus more to drizzle at the end

Directions

1. Over moderate heat in a medium pan; heat the tablespoon of oil until hot. Add & fry the pancetta until it begins to brown a little, for a couple of minutes.
2. Add the celery and carrot; gently sauté until slightly soften, for a couple of more minutes.
3. Add the zucchini, potato, tinned tomatoes, rice and water; give everything a good stir and let gently simmer until the potato is soft and rice is cooked through, for 12 to 15 minutes.
4. Add the pepper, salt & stir in the basil leaves; stir well.
5. Serve each bowl of soup with a little drizzle of garlic oil & a generous sprinkle of Parmesan.

Nutrition: Calories: 307 Carbs: 51g Fat: 7g Protein: 12g

Slow Cooker Chicken & Wild Rice Soup

Preparation Time: 15 minutes

Cooking Time: 8 hours & 35 minutes

Servings: 4

Ingredients

- 1-pound chicken breasts, boneless, skinless, cut in half
- 4 carrots, peeled & chopped
- 1 tablespoon butter
- 2 egg yolks
- ½ teaspoon dried thyme or dried herbs de Provence
- 1 bay leaf
- 4 cups chicken broth
- 1 cup water
- ¾ cup wild rice-brown rice blend
- 1 leek, small, sliced (only green parts)
- 2 teaspoon regular or garlic-infused olive oil
- 1 zucchini, large, chopped
- 3 tablespoon lemon juice (from 1 lemon)
- Black pepper and salt to taste
- For Serving:
- Freshly chopped Italian parsley
- Grated Parmesan cheese

Directions:

1. Add the entire ingredients (except olive oil, egg yolk, leek, lemon juice, black pepper, salt & the ingredients for serving) to a large slow cooker. Cook for 4 hours on high-heat or 8 hours or low-heat, until the rice is tender and chicken breasts are opaque in the thickest part. Transfer the cooked chicken breasts to a clean cutting board.
2. Now, whisk the egg yolks in a small bowl. As you whisk; slowly pour approximately ¼ cup of the hot soup into the yolks. With the slow cooker on high, pour the yolk mixture slowly into the soup; continue to stir as you pour the soup. Cover & cook for 10 minutes on high-heat.
3. Now, over medium heat in a large skillet; heat the garlic oil. Once hot; add leek, season with pepper and salt; cook for 6 to 8 minutes, until tender. Shred the chicken & add it along with the leeks to the slow cooker. Cover & cook until the chicken is just heated through, for a couple of more minutes. Feel free to add more of broth or water, if your soup is quite thick.
4. Turn off the slow cooker & stir in the lemon juice. Add some black pepper and salt to taste. Put some soup into bowls & top with fresh parsley and Parmesan.

Nutrition: Calories: 624 Carbs: 75g Fat: 17g Protein: 50g

Vegetable Soup

Prep Time: 15 minutes

Cooking Time: 60 minutes

Servings: 14

Ingredients:

- 6 cup collard greens, loosely packed, big stems removed
- 3 tablespoon tamari or low sodium soy sauce
- 1 ½ teaspoon chili powder
- 6 carrots, medium-large, sliced
- 15 ounce can diced tomatoes, salt-free
- 10 cup plus ¼ cup water
- 2 teaspoon cumin
- 6 ounces can tomato paste, salt-free
- 1 tablespoon pure maple syrup
- 3 tablespoon lemon juice
- 1 cup uncooked quinoa
- 3 teaspoon smoked paprika
- 1 tablespoon olive oil
- Black pepper & salt to taste

Directions:

1. Over moderate heat in a large cooking pot; heat the oil until hot. Add the cumin, paprika & chili powder; stir well and then add in the carrots & ¼ cup of water.

2. Cover the pot with a lid & let cook for 8 to 10 minutes, stirring every now and then. While the carrots cook; stem the greens. Stir in the remaining ingredients.
3. Increase the heat to medium-high. Cover the pot with lid again & bring everything together to a boil. Decrease the heat to medium; uncover & let simmer for 30 to 35 more minutes.

Nutrition: Calories: 78 Carbs: 15g Fat: 1g Protein: 3g

Potato & Spinach Soup

Preparation Time: 15 minutes

Cooking Time: 55 minutes

Servings: 4

Ingredients:

- 17 ounces homemade chicken stock
- A bunch of spinach; washed & sliced up
- 1 knob of ginger, finely chopped
- 5 big potatoes; peeled & cut into large cubes
- 1 teaspoon cumin powder
- 20 beans (10 green beans are low Fodmap); cut
- 1 red chili; finely chopped
- Fresh mint
- 1 stalk of celery (¼ stalk is low Fodmap); finely chopped
- Paprika
- 8 slices of lean bacon
- ½ cup tomato puree
- Sour cream

Directions:

1. Over moderate heat in a saucepan; heat a tablespoon of oil until hot & then add in the ginger mix.
2. Fry for a minute & then add cumin powder; fry for 30 more seconds.

3. Add the beans and potatoes to the ginger mix; toss for a couple of minutes, until evenly mixed.
4. Add the tomato puree and stock; cover the pan with a lid and cook until the vegetables are almost cooked through.
5. Add in the spinach & let it wilt down.
6. In the meantime; cut up the bacon into bite-sized pieces & fry in a little oil for a couple of minutes, until crisp.
7. When the spinach has blended into the soup, place approximately half of it in a food processor & carefully process on high (starting with the lowest available setting) until smooth.
8. Add pureed soup to saucepan with the remaining soup and reheat.
9. Serve in bowls & garnish each bowl with the bacon, a little sour cream, chopped mint and a sprinkling of paprika.

Nutrition: Calories: 100 Carbs: 16g Fat: 4g Protein: 2g

Carrot, Coconut and Ginger Soup

Preparation Time: 15 minutes

Cooking Time: 55 minutes

Servings: 4

Ingredients:

- 1 teaspoon turmeric
- 8 carrots
- 1 tablespoon paprika
- 4 parsnips
- 1" chunk of ginger
- 4 tablespoon coconut milk
- 1 tablespoon apple cider vinegar
- Pepper and sea salt, to taste
- 1-liter FODMAP-friendly vegetable stock or boiling water
- Toppings:
- Sunflower or pumpkin seeds

Directions:

1. Peel the ginger, parsnips and carrots & then chop into small-sized chunks.
2. Place the ginger and vegetables in a pan & add in the vegetable stock or boiling water.
3. Add in the paprika, turmeric, and pepper and salt; let simmer until vegetables are soft, for 15 to 20 minutes.

---

4. Once cooked, let the mixture to cool and then transfer it into a blender.
5. Add in the apple cider vinegar and coconut milk; blitz on high until smooth.
6. Pour the soup into bowls & top each bowl with an extra swirl of coconut milk, a handful of hemp seeds and a handful of pumpkin seeds.

Nutrition: Calories: 120 Carbs: 18g Fat: 5g Protein: 1g

Chicken Matzo Balls Soup

Preparation Time: 15 minutes

Cooking Time: 15 hours & 30 minutes

Servings: 12

Ingredients:

- For Stock:
- 1 tablespoon black peppercorns
- 3 pounds chicken wings
- 1 bay leaf
- Add any other seasonings you prefer
- 1 teaspoon parsley
- 1 tablespoon kosher salt
- For Matzo Balls:
- ½ teaspoon baking powder
- 4 eggs, large
- ½ cup olive oil
- 1 cup low-FODMAP matzo meal, gluten-free
- ½ teaspoon salt

Directions:

1. Cook the entire stock ingredients together in Crock-Pot for overnight or for 12 to 15 hours on low-heat. Let stock to cool & then strain into freezer bags.
2. For Matzo Balls: Blend the entire Matzo Balls ingredients together in a food processor until well combined.

---

3. Refrigerate until the mixture thickens, for 2 to 3 hours. Form balls from the prepared mixture.
4. Drop the prepared balls into the boiling low-FODMAP chicken stock or water.
5. Cover and let boil until plump up, for 40 minutes
6. Warm up the chicken stock again
7. Add dill weed to taste & 2 to 3 chopped carrots, if desired.
8. Just before serving, add balls to the hot soup. Garnish with fresh parsley. Serve and enjoy.

Nutrition: Calories: 190 Carbs: 0g Fat: 6g Protein: 0g

Roasted Pumpkin Soup

Preparation Time: 10 minutes

Cooking Time: 10 minutes

Servings: 1

Ingredients:

- 140g Japanese pumpkin, roasted; heated in microwave for half a minute
- 1 cup hot low FODMAP chicken stock
- 2 teaspoon chives, fresh, chopped
- Low FODMAP toast plus more of chives to garnish

Directions:

1. Put the roasted pumpkin, stock & chives in a jug; then blend using a stick blender until smooth.
2. Scoop some soup into a bowl & sprinkle with more of chives, if desired. Serve with toast.

Nutrition: Calories: 152 Carbs: 22g Fat: 3g Protein: 3g

Baked Brie with Cranberry Chutney and Caramelized Pecans

Prep Time: 15 minutes

Cooking Time: 25 minutes

Servings: 8 persons

Ingredients:

- 2 tablespoons pecans, chopped
- 1 package brie cheese with rind (8 ounce)
- 2 tablespoons packed brown sugar
- ¼ cranberry chutney
- 2 teaspoons butter, dairy-free

Directions:

1. Spray some nonstick cooking spray and preheat your oven to 350 F in advance.
2. Cut the top off the brie & place it in this dish.
3. Spread the chutney over the brie just like frosting a cake.
4. Sprinkle the top with pecans and then sprinkle with the brown sugar.
5. Dot top with the dairy-free butter.
6. Your preheated oven baked for 15 to 18 minutes, until cheese is very soft to the touch.
7. Increase the heat to 425F & bake for 5 more minutes.

8. The sugar would bubble on top and brie would start melting on the bottom. Serve with gluten free rice cakes, crackers, carrots or any of the FODMAP Free nibbles.

Nutrition: Calories: 468 Carbs: 48g Fat: 21g Protein: 19g

POULTRY AND SEAFOOD RECIPES

Coconut Shrimp

Preparation Time: 10 minutes

Cooking Time: 15 minutes

Servings: 4

Ingredients:

- 1 slice gluten-free bread, toasted
- 1/2 cup unsweetened finely shredded coconut
- 1/8 teaspoon sea salt
- 1 large egg
- 1/8 teaspoon pure vanilla extract
- 16 large raw shrimp, peeled and deveined

Directions:

1. Preheat oven to 425°F. Prepare your baking sheet with foil and coat with coconut oil spray.
2. Add toast to food processor. Pulse until fine bread crumbs form.
3. In a flat dish, mix bread crumbs with coconut and salt.
4. In a small bowl, whisk together egg and vanilla.

5. Dip each shrimp into egg mixture, then into bread-crumb/coconut mixture. Transfer to baking sheet.
6. Bake for 5 minutes. Carefully turn each shrimp over and bake for 5 minutes more or until shrimp are fully cooked through. Serve immediately.

Nutrition: Calories: 88 Fat: 5g Protein: 5g Carbohydrates: 6g

Tilapia Piccata

Preparation Time: 15 minutes

Cooking Time: 45 minutes

Servings: 6

Ingredients:

- 1/4 cup dry white wine
- 3 tablespoons freshly squeezed lemon juice
- 1 teaspoon fresh lemon zest
- 2 tablespoons capers, rinsed, drained
- 1/4 cup sweet rice flour, divided
- 1/2 teaspoon sea salt
- 1/4 teaspoon freshly ground black pepper
- 4 (6-ounce) pieces tilapia fillets
- 1 tablespoon Garlic-Infused Oil
- 1 teaspoon butter
- 1 tablespoon chopped fresh parsley

Directions:

1. In a small bowl, whisk wine, lemon juice, zest, and capers.
2. Reserve 1 teaspoon flour and set aside. Mix remaining flour with salt and pepper on a plate. Dip fish into flour.
3. Heat oil over medium heat in a large skillet. Add fish and cook 2–3 minutes per side. When fish is cooked through, remove from pan.

4. Add wine mixture and reserved flour to pan and cook 1 minute, whisking constantly. Remove from heat and stir in butter.
5. Top fish with the sauce, garnish with parsley, and serve immediately.

Nutrition: Calories: 168 Fat: 5g Protein: 23g Carbohydrates: 6g

Chinese Chicken

Preparation Time: 15 minutes

Cooking Time: 1 hour

Servings: 4

Ingredients:

- 3⁄4 cup arrowroot powder
- 1⁄2 cup white wine, divided
- 1⁄2 cup gluten-free tamari, divided
- 1 pound boneless, skinless chicken breasts, cubed
- 1⁄2 teaspoon sugar
- 1⁄2 cup Basic Roast Chicken Stock
- 2 tablespoons sesame oil, divided
- 1 teaspoon natural peanut butter
- 4 garlic cloves, peeled and slightly smashed
- 1 cup broccoli florets
- 1 cup sliced red bell pepper
- 2 cups cooked brown rice

Directions:

1. In a medium bowl, stir to combine arrowroot and 1⁄4 cup each of wine and tamari. Add chicken; stir to coat. Cover and refrigerate for 30 minutes.
2. Transfer chicken to a colander and drain marinade completely. Set chicken aside.

3. In a separate bowl, combine sugar, stock, and remaining wine and tamari.
4. In another small bowl, whisk 1 tablespoon oil and peanut butter.
5. Heat remaining oil over medium-high heat in a large wok or skillet. Add the garlic and sauté, stirring constantly, until softened and brown at the edges, about 2 minutes. Remove garlic from pan and discard, leaving oil.
6. Add chicken and stir-fry quickly, browning chicken on all sides—approximately 8–10 minutes. Scrape up and discard any loose marinade bits. Once fully cooked through, transfer chicken to a plate and cover to keep warm.
7. Add broccoli and bell pepper to skillet and quickly stir-fry for 1 minute. Add stock and peanut butter mixtures and stir. Cover, then lower heat and simmer for 5–8 minutes, until vegetables are crisp-tender.
8. Divide rice, chicken, and vegetables in their sauce evenly among four plates and serve.

Nutrition: Calories: 458 Fat: 11g Protein: 30g Carbohydrates: 53g

Caramel Oat Chicken Fingers

Preparation Time: 10 minutes

Cooking Time: 15 minutes

Servings: 4

Ingredients:

- 1 teaspoon butter
- 1 cup gluten-free rolled oats
- 1/4 teaspoon sea salt
- 1 teaspoon maple sugar
- 2 large eggs
- 1 teaspoon ground cinnamon
- 4 (3-ounce) boneless, skinless chicken breasts, pounded and cut into 1"-wide strips

Directions:

1. Heat oven to 400°F. Line a baking sheet with parchment paper and coat with coconut oil spray.
2. In a medium skillet, melt butter over medium heat. Add oats and stir. Add salt and maple sugar and stir to combine. Lower heat and stir until oats start to toast and turn light brown. Transfer oat mixture to plate to cool.
3. While oat mixture is cooling, whisk eggs in a bowl. Add cinnamon to cooled oat mixture and stir to combine.

4. Dip chicken strips in egg and then in oat mixture to fully coat all sides.
5. Put a strips on baking sheet and bake for 15–20 minutes or until chicken is fully cooked. Transfer to a platter and serve.

Nutrition: Calories: 220 Fat: 7g Protein: 24g Carbohydrates: 15g

SIDE DISHES, SAUCES AND DIPS RECIPES

Tomato Purée

Preparation Time: 5 minutes

Cooking Time: 20 minutes

Servings: 10

Ingredients:

- 1 tablespoon Garlic-Infused Oil
- 5 medium ripe tomatoes, cored, seeded, and diced
- 1 teaspoon sea salt
- 1⁄4 teaspoon freshly ground black pepper

Directions:

1. Using a large saucepan heat your oil over medium-low heat in a large saucepan. Add tomatoes to oil and stir. Season with salt and pepper. Sauté, stirring occasionally, for 15–20 minutes, until tomatoes are soft and broken down. Remove from heat to cool.
2. Put your cooled tomatoes to your food processor and then blend completely. Prepare a larger strainer over a large bowl.

3. Put your purée to a strainer. Using a large spoon strain it carefully to completely separate solids in strainer from purée in bowl.
4. Store to an airtight container and store in the refrigerator.

Nutrition: Calories: 77 Fat: 5g Protein: 2g Carbohydrates: 8g

Tomato Paste

Preparation Time: 10 minutes

Cooking Time: 2 hours

Servings: 2

Ingredients:

- 1 1/2 cups Tomato Purée

Directions:

1. Preheat oven to 300°F. Pour purée into an ovenproof skillet.
2. Cook without a cover for about 2 hours, stirring every 20 minutes, until a paste consistency is formed.
3. Cool completely.

Nutrition: Calories: 22 Fat: 0g Protein: 1g Carbohydrates: 5g

Roasted Tomato Sauce

Preparation Time: 10 minutes

Cooking Time: 25 minutes

Servings: 2

Ingredients:

- 2 tablespoons Garlic-Infused Oil
- 1 teaspoon salt
- 1 1/2 pounds fresh tomatoes, cored, seeded and diced
- 1 bay leaf
- 1/8 teaspoon crushed red pepper

Directions:

1. Preheat oven to 400°F. Line a roasting pan with parchment paper.
2. Mixed all your ingredients in a medium bowl and toss to thoroughly combine. Transfer to roasting pan and spread tomatoes in one thin layer.
3. Roast for 20 minutes, tossing halfway through. Remove and discard bay leaf. Transfer to a bowl and stir.

Nutrition: Calories: 9 Fat: 7g Protein: 1g Carbohydrates: 7g

Traditional Tomato Sauce

Preparation Time: 15 minutes

Cooking Time: 2 hours

Servings: 6

Ingredients:

- 1/4 cup extra-virgin olive oil
- 1 medium onion, peeled and quartered
- 4 garlic cloves, peeled and slightly smashed
- 11/2 cups Tomato Purée
- 1 (14-ounce) can San Marzano diced tomatoes
- 1 can whole peeled San Marzano tomatoes
- 1 teaspoon dried oregano
- 1 teaspoon dried basil
- 1 tablespoon turbinado sugar
- 1 (1" × 3") Parmesan cheese rind

Directions:

1. Using a large pan heat your oil over medium-low heat. Put the onion and garlic then sauté, stir it carefully, until your garlic is soft and brown at edges. Take it from the heat and discard onion and garlic, leaving oil.
2. Add remaining ingredients, except for cheese rind; stir to combine. Break up whole tomatoes with a pair of kitchen shears.

3. Bring to boil, then put your heat to low. Add some cheese rind and simmer uncovered, stirring occasionally, for 1½–2 hours. Remove remainder of rind before serving.

Nutrition: Calories: 180 Fat: 12g Protein: 3g Carbohydrates: 19g

Alfredo Sauce

Preparation Time: 15 minutes

Cooking Time: 20 minutes

Servings: 8

Ingredients:

- 1 tablespoon butter
- 4 garlic cloves, peeled, slightly smashed
- 1 tablespoon sweet rice flour
- 1 1/3 cups lactose-free milk
- 1 teaspoon sea salt
- 1/4 teaspoon freshly ground black pepper
- 1 cup grated Parmesan cheese
- 1/2 cup Whipped Cream

Directions:

1. Heat butter over medium-low heat in a medium saucepan. Add the garlic and sauté, stirring constantly, until softened and brown at edges. Remove and discard garlic, leaving butter.
2. Put flour and whisk constantly for 1–2 minutes until thickened and light golden brown.
3. Slowly whisk in milk. Cook, whisk it carefully, until thickened and bubbling, about 8–10 minutes. Get it from the heat, season with salt and pepper, and stir in cheese.

4. Fold in whipped cream and serve.

Nutrition: Calories: 330 Fat: 24g Protein: 17g Carbohydrates: 11g

SNACKS, DESSERT AND APPETIZER RECIPES

Low Carb No-Bake Nutty Caramel Energy Bites

Preparation Time: 5 minutes

Cooking Time: 0 minute

Servings: 10

Ingredients:

- ½ cup raw walnuts
- ½ cup raw pecans
- ½ cup cashews
- 1 Date pitted
- 1 Tablespoon + 1 teaspoon virgin coconut oil
- 1 Tablespoon + 1 teaspoon pure maple syrup
- 1 Teaspoon pure vanilla extract
- ¼ teaspoon fine sea salt
- Optional pumpkin pie spice and/or hemp seeds for coating

Directions:

-

1. Join all fixings, with the exception of discretionary pumpkin pie zest and hemp seeds, in a nourishment processor. Heartbeat fixings, scratching sides of the nourishment processor as fundamental, until all around joined and nuts are all around finely cleaved without going in to nut margarine.
2. Structure blend into 10 ~ 1-inch balls. Coat with discretionary pumpkin pie flavor or potentially hemp seeds whenever wanted and store in icebox or cooler until prepared to eat.

Nutrition: Calories: 269 Carbs: 31g Fat: 15g Protein: 7g

Low FODMAP Chocolate Pavlova with Pomegranate, Raspberries & Kiwi

Preparation Time: 20 minutes

Cooking Time: 2 hours

Servings: 8

Ingredients:

- Meringue:
- 4 Ounces (115 g) bittersweet chocolate, finely chopped, preferably at least 60 to 70% cacao
- 4 Large egg whites
- ¼ teaspoon cream of tartar
- 1 Cup (198 g) sugar, preferably superfine
- 2 teaspoons cornstarch
- ½ teaspoon apple cider vinegar
- ½ teaspoon vanilla extract
- Topping:
- 1 Cup (240 ml) heavy cream, chilled
- 2 Teaspoons confectioners' sugar
- 3 Tablespoons pomegranate seeds
- 12 Raspberries, very firm and fresh
- 2 Green kiwi, peeled and sliced crosswise into thin rounds

Directions:

1. For the Meringue: Preheat broiler to 250°F/121°C. Line a preparing sheet field with material paper and follow a 9-inch (23 cm) hover on the paper; turn paper over.

2. Dissolve the chocolate until easy and allow to chill to scarcely heat; installed a safe spot.

3. In a great, oil-free bowl whip egg whites with inflatable whip connection of stand blender or utilize an electric powered mixer on low speed till foamy. Include cream of tartar and hold beating, going tempo to high, till delicate pinnacles shape. Include sugar slowly and beat till meringue is hardened and reflexive so that you can take a few minutes. Beat in cornstarch, vinegar, and vanilla.

4. Sprinkle the chocolate over the meringue and in all respects tenderly make more than one folds to deliver chocolate streaks in the course of the meringue. You can OVER blend in all respects effectively. Decide in want of much less.

5. Scoop the meringue onto fabric inside the circle and make use of the returned of a giant spoon to assist shape a spherical plate in the drawn circle, being aware so as not to exhaust the marbling. Make a moderate sorrow inside the focal factor of the circle. You will hear the whipped cream and natural product inside the middle and a downturn within the meringue will assist hold the fixings.

6. A spot in stove and heat for 1 hour 15 minutes, at that point, test the meringue circle. It ought to be sparkling, dry and simply tinged with the faintest degree of

shading. Keep heating for 15 minutes more if essential. Mood killer stove and enable the plate to chill inside the broiler. Once cooled, the plate is probably put away in a water/air evidence compartment at room temperature for as long as 3 days.

7. For the Toppings:

8. Whip the cream in a clean and calm bowl with the sugar until the shape of a touchy pinnacle. Spot meringue circle on level presentation platter. Heap the whipped cream inside the focal point of the meringue, permitting a fringe of meringue to stay. Spot natural product over whipped cream, to a wonderful quantity, and serve in (chaotic) wedges with spoons to scoop the whole thing up.

Nutrition: Calories: 314 Carbs: 44g Protein: 3g Fat: 10g

No Bake Cocoa Lemon Energy Bites & Cocoa Lemon Truffles

Preparation Time: 8 minutes

Cooking Time: 0 minute

Servings: 10

Ingredients:

- Energy Bites AND Truffles
- 1 Cup pecans
- 2 Tablespoons cocoa powder
- 2 Tablespoons pure maple syrup
- 2 Teaspoons lemon juice
- 1 Teaspoon lemon zest
- 1 - Teaspoon ground cinnamon
- ¼ teaspoon pure vanilla extract
- 1/8 teaspoon sea salt
- Energy Bites
- ½ cup gluten-free oats
- For Truffles
- 1/3 cup pecans additional
- 3 Tablespoons Hempseeds

Directions:

1. Join all fixings in a nourishment processor, and procedure until the blend is sticky and all around consolidated.

2. Shape blend into 10 ~ 1-inch balls, and spot-on a plate or plate fixed with material paper. You can eat them quickly, or place them in the cooler for in any event 10 minutes

Nutrition: Calories: 110 Carbs: 10g Protein: 2g Fat: 8g

Pesto Chicken Wings

Preparation Time: 20 minutes

Cooking Time: 55 minutes

Servings: 12 persons

Ingredients:

- 2 ½ to 3 pounds chicken wings, made up of drumettes & flats
- ¼ cup long shred Parmesan cheese
- 1 ½ cups Basil Pesto, divided
- Freshly ground black pepper & kosher salt to taste

Directions:

1. Line a large-sized rimmed sheet pan with the aluminum foil and then coat the foil with nonstick spray and preheat your oven to 400 F in advance.
2. Put the wings in a large bowl & season them generously with pepper and lightly with salt. Add approximately ¾ of the pesto; toss well until evenly coated. Place the pesto-coated wings on the prepared pan & roast in the preheated oven until the wings are just cooked through, for 35 to 45 minutes.
3. Remove the pan from oven & brush the leftover pesto over the wings. Sprinkle with cheese; serve immediately and enjoy.

Nutrition: Calories: 245 Carbs: 3g Fat: 0g Protein: 39g

Deviled Eggs

Preparation Time: 20 minutes

Cooking Time: 30 minutes

Servings: 24 persons

Ingredients:

- 12 hard-boiled eggs, large, peeled & cut lengthwise
- ⅛ Teaspoon cayenne pepper
- Chives, chopped
- 1 tablespoon Dijon mustard
- ½ cup mayonnaise
- Salt, paprika and pepper, to taste

Directions:

1. Remove the cooked yolks carefully & place them in a large bowl. Using a large fork; mash the yolks well. Add mustard with mayonnaise & cayenne; stir until completely smooth. Season with pepper and salt.
2. Put your egg whites with the prepared yolk mixture. Top with chives and paprika. Serve chilled & enjoy.

Nutrition: Calories: 150 Carbs: 0g Fat: 4g Protein: 6g

Dark Chocolate and Raspberry Brownies

Preparation Time: 15 minutes

Cooking Time: 30 minutes

Servings: 10 pieces

Ingredients:

- 1 cup of dairy-free butter
- 1 cup of dark chocolate
- 1 cup of brown sugar
- 4 egg-whites
- 1 cup of all-purpose flour
- 4 tablespoons of dark cocoa powder
- 1 tablespoon of xanthan gum
- ¾ cup of raspberries
- Chopped walnuts for topping

Directions:

1. Prepare to preheat your oven to 350 degrees F (180 C).
2. Bring a large pot of water to a boil.
3. Place a large microwave bowl over the pot.
4. Add dairy-free butter, chocolate and brown sugar to the bowl. Keep stirring until all the ingredients melt.
5. When your mixture is smooth, remove it from the heat and add the egg-whites. Whisk well by using a hand blender.

---

6. Using another bowl, combine the flour, cocoa powder and xanthan gum. Mix well.
7. Slowly pour the flour mixture into the chocolate mixture and mix well using a spoon. Make sure there are no lumps.
8. Lightly fold in the raspberries and pour the mixture into a prepared baking tray. Sprinkle chopped walnuts on top.
9. Bake the brownies for about 30 minutes.
10. Let your brownies cool for 15 minutes before cutting.
11. Serve warm.

Nutrition: Calories: 182 Carbs: 16g Fat: 13g Protein: 4g

Blueberry Crumble Slice

Preparation Time: 15 minutes

Cooking Time: 30 minutes

Servings: 10 slices

Ingredients:

- For the base
- 2 ½ cups of self-rising flour
- ¼ teaspoon of salt
- ½ teaspoon of ground cinnamon
- ¾ cup of white sugar
- 1 cup of dairy-free butter
- 1 egg-white
- For the filling
- 2 1/2 cups of blueberries
- 3 teaspoons of corn flour
- ¼ cup of white sugar

Directions:

1. Ready to preheat the oven to 350 degrees F (180 C).
2. Prepare a medium-sized baking sheet or tray with some dairy-free butter and set aside.
3. In a bowl, combine the self-rising flour with the salt, cinnamon powder and ¾ cup of sugar. Mix well using your hands. The mixture should be slightly crumbly.

4. Melt the dairy-free butter and pour that into the flour mixture.
5. Crack an egg into the bowl and use your hands to knead the mixture into a firm dough.
6. Take half of the dough and spread it evenly at the bottom of the pan.
7. Add the blueberries as the next layer.
8. In a small bowl, combine the corn flour with the ¼ cup of sugar and sprinkle that on top of the blueberries.
9. Your second half of your dough should crumble for the blueberries.
10. Bake for 30 minutes until the crust is nice and golden.
11. Cool for 15 minutes.
12. Slice and serve.

Nutrition: Calories: 311 Carbs: 63g Fat: 7g Protein: 2g

Carrot and Chocolate Bundtlets

Preparation Time: 20 minutes

Cooking Time: 20 minutes

Servings: 4

Ingredients:

- ¼ cup of almond milk
- 2 tablespoons of virgin coconut oil
- 1 medium carrot, pureed
- ¼ cup of brown sugar
- 1 ½ tablespoon of cocoa powder
- ½ cup of rice flour
- 1 teaspoon of baking powder
- For candied almonds
- Around 10 almonds, roughly chopped
- 1 tablespoon of maple syrup or honey
- ½ teaspoon of ground cinnamon

Directions:

1. Ready to preheat the oven to 350 degrees F (180 C).
2. Prepare 4 small-sized baking molds with dairy-free butter and set aside.
3. In a large bowl, combine the almond milk with the coconut oil, carrot puree and sugar. Whisk using a blender.

4. Slowly add the rice flour and fold it in using a spoon. Always check that your mixture has no lumps.
5. Add the cocoa and baking powder. Mix again.
6. Fill the muffin molds about halfway up with this batter. Set aside.
7. Put a parchment paper on a flat microwave dish.
8. Combine the almonds with the maple syrup and ground cinnamon and spread that mixture over the dish.
9. Place the muffin molds and the tray with the almonds in the oven and bake for 15 minutes.
10. Remove the almonds and allow the cakes to bake for 10 more minutes.
11. Take the cakes out of the molds, top them with almond candies and serve.

Nutrition: Calories: 225 Carbs: 20g Fat: 15g Protein: 3g

Gluten Free Carrot Soufflé

Preparation Time: 20 minutes

Cooking Time: 20 minutes

Servings: 8

Ingredients

- 2 pounds carrots
- ¾ cup of sugar
- 1 ½ teaspoons of baking powder
- 1 ½ teaspoons of vanilla extract
- ½ teaspoon of cinnamon
- ¼ teaspoon of nutmeg
- ¼ teaspoon of ground black pepper
- 2 heaping tablespoons of gluten-free flour
- 3 egg-whites
- ½ cup of dairy-free butter, softened
- 2 tablespoons of grated carrot for topping
- 2 tablespoons of icing sugar for topping

Directions:

1. Ready to preheat the oven to 350 degrees F (180 C).
2. Wash, peel and dice the carrots.
3. Fill a large pot with 2-3 cups of water. Bring the water to a boil and add the carrots to it.
4. Cover the pot and cook the carrots until they are tender (about 5 minutes).

5. Once they cool down, drain the excess water and add them to a blender.
6. Add the sugar, baking powder, vanilla, cinnamon, nutmeg and pepper.
7. To obtained a smooth paste blend it well and transfer to a bowl.
8. Mix in the flour, eggs and softened dairy-free butter.
9. Pour your mixture to the prepared baking tray and bake for about an hour. You want the top to be golden brown.
10. Top with icing sugar and grated carrots.

Nutrition: Calories: 400 Carbs: 30g Fat: 10g Protein: 5g

Low FODMAP Coconut Chiffon Spice Cake

Preparation Time: 20 minutes

Cooking Time: 60 minutes

Servings: 12

Ingredients:

- 3 cups of all-purpose flour
- ½ teaspoon of baking soda
- 1 teaspoon of baking powder
- ½ teaspoon of salt
- ½ teaspoon of ground nutmeg
- 1 tablespoon of xanthan gum
- ¼ teaspoon of clove powder
- 2 cups of sugar
- 5 tablespoons of dairy-free butter
- 6 egg-whites and yolks
- 2 teaspoons of almond extract
- 2 teaspoons of vanilla extract
- 1 cup of virgin coconut oil
- 1 cup of coconut milk
- ¾ cup of desiccated coconut

Directions:

1. Ready to preheat the oven to 350 degrees F (180 C).
2. Prepare a baking tray with cooking spray.

3. In a bowl, combine the all-purpose flour with the baking soda, baking powder, and salt, nutmeg powder, xanthan gum and clove powder. Mix well.

4. In another bowl, combine the sugar with the dairy-free butter. Whisk using a blender until it becomes nice and fluffy.

5. Separate the egg yolks from the egg whites. Keep both.

6. Whisk the egg yolks with a blender until they are frothy.

7. Add almond extract, vanilla extract and coconut oil to the yolk mixture. Mix well.

8. Now use the blender to whisk the egg-whites until you see soft peaks.

9. Pour the yolk mixture into the flour mixture slowly while adding the coconut milk. Whisk slightly using the blender.

10. Gently fold the desiccated coconut and egg-whites into the batter.

11. Pour the batter into the prepared tin.

12. Bake for 45 to 50 minutes and allow it to cool on a rack for the 15 minutes.

13. Slice and serve and you can store in an airtight container for up to 7 days.

Nutrition: Calories: 208 Carbs: 29g Fat: 8g Protein: 4g

DRINKS RECIPES

Breakfast Smoothie

Preparation Time: 5 minutes

Cooking Time: 5 minutes

Servings: 1

Ingredients:

- 1 tablespoon rolled oats
- 1 cup almond milk
- 1 banana, small
- A good pinch of ground cinnamon
- 1 heaped teaspoon flaxseed

Directions

1. Place the entire ingredients together in a blender; blend on high (starting with the lowest possible settings) until completely smooth.
2. Serve immediately and enjoy.

Nutrition: Calories: 190 Carbs: 34g Fat: 3g Protein: 6g

Banana Peanut Butter Smoothie

Preparation Time: 5 minutes

Cooking Time: 5 minutes

Servings: 2

Ingredients:

- 1 cup yogurt, lactose-free
- 2 tablespoons peanut butter
- 1 medium banana, frozen, peeled
- 2 teaspoons chia seeds
- ¼ teaspoon vanilla extract

Directions:

1. Add chia seeds to a dry blender; pulse on high for a couple of minutes, until you get powder like consistency. Turn the blender off & scrape the sides down using a spatula & gather the chia seed powder to the bottom.
2. Add frozen banana chunks, yogurt, vanilla, and peanut butter. Blend on high again for a minute. Stop & scrape down the blender, moving any chunks that did not blend. Cover & pulse again for a couple of more seconds, until completely smooth.

Nutrition: Calories: 303 Carbs: 45g Fat: 9g Protein: 16g

Chocolate Strawberry Smoothie

Preparation Time: 5 minutes

Cooking Time: 5 minutes

Servings: 1

Ingredients:

- 1 banana, small, frozen
- ⅛ Cup peanut or seed butter
- 1 cup milk, any of your favorite
- 2 tablespoon high quality cocoa powder
- ½ cup strawberries
- 1 tablespoon Chia seeds
- A dash of sea salt

Directions:

1. Place the entire ingredients together in a blender; blend on high until completely smooth.
2. Serve immediately and enjoy.

Nutrition: Calories: 264 Carbs: 40g Fat: 7g Protein: 11g

Chocolate Mocha Smoothie

Preparation Time: 5 minutes

Cooking Time: 5 minutes

Servings: 1

Ingredients:

- 1 frozen banana, sliced into pieces
- 10 gr peanut butter
- 1 tablespoon cacao powder
- 175 ml unsweetened almond milk
- 1 double espresso

Directions:

1. Place the entire ingredients together in a blender; blend on high until completely smooth.
2. Pour the mixture in a large glass (with a straw). Serve immediately and enjoy.

Nutrition: Calories: 300 Carbs: 7g Fat: 4g Protein: 30g